Beyond Trash

Rethinking Waste in the Modern World

Ella Stayton

Table of contents

Introduction

"Beyond Trash" stands out as an insightful reference that looks deeply into the complicated tapestry of trash management in an era of increased environmental awareness and altering paradigms of consumerism. The multiple facets of garbage and its enormous ramifications for our world and communities are made clear to readers in this engaging text, which transcends conventional viewpoints.

As "Beyond Trash" explores the fields of environmental science, social equality, economics, and innovation, viewers can expect a comprehensive investigation of the complex web of waste management practices. The book peels back the layers of waste management to reveal its unintended repercussions via a rich combination of well-researched analyses, fascinating stories, and thought-provoking case studies. The book carefully reveals the complexity that underpins garbage's presence in our lives, from the widespread environmental effects of landfill emissions and plastic contamination to the social gaps worsened by poor waste disposal. The documentary "Beyond Trash" offers fascinating peeks into transformational technology, neighborhood projects, and regulatory changes that are altering our relationship with garbage, serving as a beacon of hope rather than just exposing problems.

The ability of "Beyond Trash" to smoothly combine academic rigor with understandable writing makes it the best resource available on the topic. The book, written by a specialist in waste management, environmental science, sociology, and economics, draws on their combined knowledge to give a thorough yet comprehensible analysis of trash-related problems. The book is approachable to a wide audience, from students and academics to politicians and concerned citizens, thanks to the inclusion of real-world situations and creative solutions. Beyond rubbish" offers helpful suggestions, instilling a sense of urgency and enabling readers to take an active role in the expanding story of rubbish management in the modern world. It does more than just identify the problems we confront. "Beyond Trash" justifiably asserts its place as the go-to resource for anybody wishing to sort through the intricacies of trash management and plot a sustainable route for the future as a tribute to its unmatched research and forward-looking perspective.

What is waste management?

Waste management encompasses the complex process of coordinating cultural attitudes, technical approaches, and legislative frameworks to appropriately deal with the byproducts of human consumption. It goes beyond the everyday task of getting rid of undesirable things. By limiting their production, maximizing their reuse, recycling, or conversion into useful resources, and finally guaranteeing their safe and sustainable disposal, wasted materials may have a positive influence on the environment, society, and the economy. Waste management, in its simplest form, is the proactive effort to reframe our relationship with things we no longer find useful, turning them from a burden on the environment and society into a tactical opportunity for conservation and regeneration.

I've decided to write a thorough book that goes beyond the idea of trash management as we know it today. In "Rethinking Waste," I set out on a quest to unravel the complexity of waste management, exploring its antecedents, current issues, and potential futures. Beyond the mechanics, this book will examine the cultural, psychological, and ethical aspects of trash management, shedding light on how our interaction with garbage affects our identities as consumers and environmental stewards. This book intends to inspire a paradigm change that reframes waste management as a common duty for a sustainable future by fusing tales of innovation, policy development, and community participation.

Chapter One

The Hidden Impact of Waste

Waste, which includes a variety of products abandoned after their intended use, is sometimes seen as an unavoidable result of human activity. While it is well-accepted that trash has apparent effects such as overflowing landfills and contaminated seas, there is a complex web of hidden effects that influence ecosystems, economies, and communities. This article explores the waste's diverse repercussions while underlining its often underappreciated impacts on the economic, social, and environmental spheres.

- **Environmental impacts**

Waste has significant negative effects on the ecosystem in addition to surface-level pollution and landscape damage. The greenhouse gas emissions produced during garbage breakdown are one of the hidden effects. Methane, an extremely strong greenhouse gas that contributes to global warming, is produced by organic waste in landfills. Plastics' long-term persistence in the environment, which may endure for millennia, disturbs ecosystems as the microplastics they produce seep into terrestrial and aquatic settings and harm both aquatic and terrestrial life. In addition, resource depletion and habitat damage are exacerbated by the mining and manufacturing of raw materials to replace discarded items. Increased energy and water use during industrial processes is one of the indirect environmental effects of waste, which feeds the cycle of resource exploitation.

- **Societal Impacts**

Waste's covert social effects ripple across underserved areas, exacerbating socioeconomic disparities. Poor waste management disproportionately impacts vulnerable communities, exposing them to dangerous chemicals and resulting in negative health repercussions. Informal garbage pickers, who are often found in underdeveloped nations, are exposed to work dangers and health concerns when collecting recyclables from landfills and dumps. Additionally, the aesthetics of neighborhoods are impacted by the visual blight brought on by poorly managed waste sites, which lowers property prices and lowers people's quality of life in general. This may lead to a poor impression of the place and hinder both community cohesiveness and economic growth.

- **Financial Impacts**

Even while waste management requires money, trash's hidden economic effects go well beyond simple management expenses. Resource waste has serious economic ramifications because landfills lose valuable resources that may be recovered or used in new ways. By doing this, a linear economic paradigm is maintained rather than a more sustainable circular economy.

Additionally, the financial burden of medical expenses resulting from diseases linked to waste falls heavily on both the public and private sectors. Industries are under pressure due to the depletion of natural resources brought on by the rise in demand for raw materials, which might cause supply chain disruptions and price fluctuations.

The Changing Landscape of Waste

In the 21st century, the landscape of waste management is undergoing a profound transformation, driven by a confluence of technological advancements, evolving consumer behaviors, and growing environmental consciousness. The traditional linear model of "take, make, dispose" is gradually giving way to a circular paradigm that emphasizes reduction, reuse, and recycling.

- **Technological Advancements**

Advancements in technology are catalyzing a seismic shift in waste management practices. Smart waste management systems, equipped with sensors and data analytics, are revolutionizing waste collection and disposal. These systems optimize collection routes, reduce operational costs, and minimize environmental impact by ensuring that waste is collected only when necessary.

Moreover, emerging technologies like artificial intelligence (AI) and machine learning are enhancing waste sorting and recycling processes. AI-powered robots can efficiently sort and separate different types of recyclables, improving recycling rates and reducing contamination. These technologies also facilitate the identification of hazardous materials and allow for better tracking of waste flows, enabling more effective regulation and accountability.

- **Evolving Consumer Behaviors**

Changing consumer behaviors are playing a pivotal role in reshaping the waste landscape. As awareness about the environmental impact of waste grows, consumers are increasingly demanding sustainable products and packaging. This shift has prompted companies to explore alternatives such as biodegradable packaging, reusable containers, and minimalistic designs that reduce waste at the source. The rise of the sharing economy and collaborative consumption further influences waste generation. Peer-to-peer platforms for renting and sharing items reduce the need for ownership and the subsequent disposal of rarely used goods. This not only decreases the volume of waste but also encourages a shift towards a more sustainable lifestyle.

- **Challenges and Opportunities**

While the changing landscape of waste management holds immense promise, it is not without its challenges. The complex and global nature of supply chains makes it difficult to ensure responsible waste management throughout the product lifecycle. E-waste, for example, poses challenges due to its toxic components and international trade complexities. Additionally, the transition to new waste management approaches requires investment in infrastructure, public awareness campaigns, and regulatory frameworks. The lack of consistent policies and harmonized regulations across different regions can impede progress. Moreover, ensuring inclusivity and equitable distribution of benefits from these changes is essential to prevent further marginalization of vulnerable communities.

Consequences of Traditional Waste Management

The mainstay of managing society's trash has long been traditional waste management, which emerged from a linear consumption model. However, this strategy has far-reaching effects that go beyond simple collecting and disposal. This book explores the hidden and sometimes disregarded effects of conventional waste management methods, illuminating their long-term effects on the environment, society, and the economy.

Traditional waste management has unintended repercussions that go beyond the practices used on the surface and have an impact on the ecological, social, and economic domains. There is an urgent need for reevaluation due to the linear model's disregard for the environment's limited capacity and the social effects of improper waste management.

A sustainable option is to move towards a circular economy, which emphasizes lowering waste production, reusing goods, and recycling resources. Governments, businesses, and people must work together to adopt efficient waste reduction programs, enhance recycling technology, and encourage responsible consumption to adapt to this paradigm shift.

We have the chance to restructure our relationship with resources, reduce ecological damage, address social inequities, and promote economic resilience by addressing the hidden effects of conventional waste management. We all share responsibility for moving towards sustainable waste management, which has the power to turn our current problems into a time of balance and harmony.

The Need for a Waste Management Paradigm Shift

The urgent need for a fundamental paradigm change in waste management systems cannot be stressed at a time marked by increasing environmental issues and the unrelenting acceleration of resource use. The need for change is clear in the environmental, social, and economic spheres and necessitates a firm break with tradition.

- **Environmental Imperatives**

Traditional waste management methods have obvious ecological consequences, including pollution, resource depletion, and climate change. Waste is carelessly dumped in landfills, which significantly increases greenhouse gas emissions and worsens global warming. We must change from this unsustainable course to one based on a circular economy that reduces waste production, increases resource recovery, and reduces emissions. Stringent action is required to minimize plastic waste production, improve recycling capabilities, and promote biodegradable alternatives due to the ongoing expansion of plastic garbage, which causes irreparable damage to ecosystems and marine life.

- **Social and Equity Imperatives**

Equity issues highlight how urgent it is to reform waste management. Where landfills and other waste facilities are often located, marginalized populations bear a disproportionately heavy cost from trash's negative effects. The higher health risks and worse quality of life in these places exacerbate socioeconomic disparities. Social justice concerns must be included in waste management plans as a result of a paradigm shift to ensure that the costs and rewards of sustainable practices are spread fairly. Communities might feel more invested in and engaged in the transformational process by being educated about and involved in trash reduction projects.

- **Economic Imperatives**

There are several financial costs associated with poor waste management. Municipalities struggle with the rising expenses of managing landfills, collecting garbage, and disposing of it. By promoting circular economies, where trash is used as a resource rather than a burden, a paradigm shift provides the possibility of economic resilience. In addition to lowering waste-related expenses, investing in recycling infrastructure, innovation, and green technology also creates new opportunities for sustainable economic development and job creation.

The environmental, social, and economic realities of the contemporary world need a paradigm change in waste management at this critical juncture. To move away from the linear paradigm of garbage disposal and towards a circular, sustainable future, immediate action is needed. Strong regulatory frameworks, technical advancements, and collective accountability from organizations, businesses, and people are required for this. The moment for change has arrived, and accepting it is not an option but rather a need to ensure a prosperous and peaceful future for future generations.

Chapter Two

Understanding Modern Waste Generation

The complexities of modern trash creation are inextricably linked to the dynamics of changing production, consumption, and lifestyle choices in today's society. At its heart, it stands for the outward expression of our society's norms and reflects the interaction of several elements, from technology development to cultural transformations. A new age of electronic waste has been brought about by the explosion of consumer electronics and short-lived items, while our dependence on consumables with high levels of convenience is mirrored by the explosive growth of packing materials. Modern trash includes not just the tangible things we throw away but also the social and ecological myths that guide our resource-use behaviors.

Analyzing this complex environment reveals that the growth of throwaway culture and intentional obsolescence have a key role in the rising flood of garbage. Due to their enduring presence in landfills and seas, single-use plastics have come to represent contemporary garbage. The rise of e-waste, which is defined as abandoned devices that often include dangerous materials, is also notable. Waste creation rises along with economies and urbanization because of rising consumer demand for goods and services. Examining the complex web of components, such as consumer behavior, industry practices, technology innovation, and regulatory frameworks, is necessary to comprehend contemporary waste creation.

Understanding contemporary trash creation goes beyond numerical measures to include a deeper understanding of the psychological, cultural, and economic foundations that drive this phenomenon in an age of increased environmental consciousness and the knowledge of limited resources. Such comprehension is crucial for guiding our trajectory towards more sustainable practices and supporting the creation of comprehensive waste management plans that are compatible with our modern environment.

Exploring the Sources of Waste in the 21st Century

The sources of garbage in the 21st century's dynamic environment have changed, reflecting the complex interactions between socioeconomic, consumer, and technical trends. This investigation dives further into the many sources of garbage in the modern day, shedding light on the many components that weave together to form the intricate web of waste creation.

- **Consumerism and Disposable Culture**

The rise in trash output is mostly due to consumerism, which is supported by marketing techniques that emphasize novelty and a feeling of urgency. An age of single-use things has arrived because of the culture of disposability, which is motivated by a need for ease and rapid pleasure. This tendency is best shown by the widespread usage of single-use plastics in packaging, bottles, and bags. These items, which are intended for transient usage, amass quickly in landfills and seas, creating a long-lasting environmental mark. Additionally, the dilemma caused by electronic trash (also known as "e-waste") is exacerbated by the practice of planned obsolescence, in which items are purposefully made to have a short lifetime. Smartphones, computers, and other electronic devices rapidly become old, requiring regular replacements and forcing the dumping of functioning but "outdated" items.

- **Industrial Processes and Manufacturing Byproducts**

Due to the size and complexity of contemporary production processes, industrialization, a defining feature of the 21st century, is a substantial source of waste. Large-scale consequences of mass production sometimes pose a problem for conventional waste management techniques. These byproducts might be extra materials thrown away during manufacturing or chemical waste in the form of contaminants. For instance, the fashion business adds to waste by discarding of unsold items, fabric remnants, and the quick change of trends. Similar to how the popularity of fast-moving consumer goods (FMCG) causes a large amount of packaging waste to be produced. Packaging trash, which includes anything from plastic wrappers to non-recyclable materials, has come to represent the difficulties presented by the current garbage environment.

- **E-Waste and Technological Innovation**

Despite being transformational, technological advancement has created a new kind of garbage known as "e-waste." Electronic equipment quickly became obsolete due to the fast pace of invention. Older devices are often thrown away without suitable recycling procedures in place as customers hurry to get the newest technology. E-waste includes appliances, computers, and their parts in addition to gadgets. If not properly handled, the hazardous compounds included in these goods, such as heavy metals and toxic chemicals, pose threats to the environment and human health.

- **Cultural Shifts and Lifestyle Impact**

Waste creation is significantly impacted by cultural changes and evolving lifestyles. Fast fashion creates an increasing quantity of textile waste due to the quick turnover of fashion trends. Clothing that is still wearable gets discarded in favor of new styles that are more reasonably priced. Aside from that, the digital era has given birth to intangible garbage, such as e-waste in the form of deleted online accounts, obsolete digital data, and abandoned websites. These trash types demonstrate the need to expand the definition of waste beyond tangible objects to include digital and virtual spaces as well.

In conclusion, investigating the origins of garbage in the twenty-first century reveals a rich tapestry of elements that interact to form our waste environment. Industrialization, consumerism, technical advancement, and cultural dynamics all play complex roles in trash production. To develop comprehensive waste management plans that meet the particular problems of our day, advance sustainable practices, and strike the right balance between development and environmental stewardship, it is essential to comprehend these sources holistically.

Quantifying the Scale of the Problem of Waste Management

The size of the waste management problem has reached historic levels as we go through the twenty-first century, endangering both the environment's sustainability and human well-being. To fully appreciate the scope of this problem, it is necessary to examine the startling numbers and complex processes that underpin garbage creation, disposal, and its far-reaching effects.

- **The Vast Landscape of Waste Generation**

Understanding the enormous amount of garbage produced worldwide is the first step in quantifying the scope of the waste management issue. Over 2 billion metric tonnes of municipal solid garbage are produced globally each year, according to the World Bank, with that amount expected to rise by 70% by 2050 if present trends continue. This diagram only represents a section of the waste ecosystem since it does not include difficulties posed by hazardous waste, industrial wastes, and electronic trash (often known as "e-waste"). This problem is made worse by the expansion of urban populations and consumption-driven economies, which causes trash production to outpace the infrastructure for disposal now in place.

• Effects on Health and Ecosystems

The implications for ecology and health provide a striking reflection of the scope of the waste management problem. Poor waste management and disposal procedures contaminate soil and water, which causes a variety of environmental problems. For instance, plastics, which make up a significant portion of contemporary garbage, are renowned for persisting in the environment; each year, 8 million metric tonnes of plastic enter the ocean. This buildup threatens aquatic life, disturbs marine ecosystems, and may even result in human consumption of microplastics through the food chain. Additionally, the open burning of garbage degrades the air quality and poses a health risk to the public, especially in low-income neighborhoods close to waste disposal facilities.

- **Social and Economic Costs**

The size of waste management is quantified, including the social and economic costs. Governments and municipalities spend a lot of money on waste management-related expenses including collection, transport, and disposal. As garbage quantities rise, these expenses are predicted to skyrocket. Additionally, the issue is made worse by the hidden expenses of healthcare associated with diseases caused by waste as well as the loss of potential economic value owing to inefficient resource use. Socially marginalized populations suffer the most from poor waste management techniques since they are more likely to experience health concerns, decreased property values, and social stigmatization.

Chapter Three

Innovative Approaches

The need to reevaluate waste management has sparked a surge of creative solutions that go against accepted wisdom and open the door to a future that is resource- and sustainably wiser. In this discourse, we explore cutting-edge waste management innovation and examine cutting-edge tactics that are changing how we see, handle, and reuse waste materials.

- **Circular Economy Paradigm**

The circular economy is a paradigm shift that seeks to reduce waste by reinventing goods, materials, and processes. It is at the core of creative waste management. The circular economy promotes closed-loop systems where things are made to be durable, repairable, and recyclable as opposed to the linear "take, make, dispose" approach. Businesses are starting to use this strategy by creating goods that are simple to dismantle so that their parts may be recycled or used for something else. This strategy not only saves waste but also decreases the requirement for virgin materials, supporting sustainability across sectors.

- **Zero Waste Initiatives**

As a comprehensive plan to reduce trash output, the "zero waste" movement has gained traction. The goal is to divert garbage away from landfills and incinerator plants, from small businesses to big families. The goal is to send as little residual trash as possible to disposal facilities by aggressive waste reduction, composting, and recycling initiatives. Utilizing cutting-edge waste-to-energy technology, organic waste is transformed into electricity or biogas, decreasing the need for fossil fuels and minimizing the effects of waste decomposition.

- **Technological Innovations**

Technology has become a potent ally in the effort to redefine waste management. Sensors, data analytics, and real-time monitoring are used by smart waste management systems to optimize garbage collection routes, save fuel costs, and boost operational effectiveness. Robotics and artificial intelligence are used in advanced sorting systems to precisely separate recyclable items from mixed waste streams, increasing recycling rates and reducing contamination. In addition, blockchain technology is being investigated to increase supply chain transparency for trash, guarantee correct disposal, and monitor hazardous waste.

- **Upcycling and Creative Reuse**

Upcycling, a concept that entails transforming waste materials into goods of greater value, is encouraging innovation in waste management. Waste materials like tires, plastic bottles, and shipping containers are being repurposed by designers, artists, and inventors into beautiful and useful objects. With this strategy, trash is not only kept out of landfills but also the untapped potential of discarded materials is brought to light.

Together, these cutting-edge strategies are defining a new era in waste management, one where environmental stewardship, resource efficiency, and sustainability are prioritized in decision-making. These creative approaches beg us to reimagine our relationship with garbage and create a world where waste is no longer a problem but rather a possible solution as we approach a more responsible future.

A crucial step towards balancing our contemporary way of life with the planet's limited resources is adopting the circular economy. The paradigm change from linear to circular systems has the power to completely alter how we generate, consume, and dispose of waste. It represents a shift away from a throwaway mentality towards one that values resource efficiency, recycles resources and respects the bounds of the world. We have the chance to construct a path toward sustainability, resilience, and a future that thrives within the confines of our linked world by realigning our practices with the principles of the circular economy.

Case Studies: Successful Models of Waste Reduction and Management

Sweden is home to one of the best cases of efficient waste management and reduction. Sweden's waste management system serves as an example for other nations since it is effective and environmentally friendly. The nation has made outstanding progress in reducing waste and increasing resource recovery.

The success story of waste reduction in Sweden is a result of several regulations, technology, and campaigns to raise awareness among the general people. The nation has established a comprehensive strategy that emphasizes waste reduction, reuse, recycling, and energy recovery. Their substantial waste-to-energy (WTE) program is one of the major elements. In Sweden, almost 50% of household garbage is burned to provide heat and electricity, which powers hundreds of thousands of households and lessens reliance on fossil fuels.

In addition to waste-to-energy, recycling is highly valued in Sweden. The nation has put in place a strict system of garbage sorting that encourages people to segregate their trash into several categories including plastics, paper, glass, and organic waste. People may easily engage in recycling activities because of the effective garbage collection infrastructure, which includes frequent collections and well-positioned recycling facilities.

Sweden's dedication to reducing landfill consumption is yet another noteworthy facet of its achievement in waste management. Less than 1% of the nation's total garbage is dumped in landfills, hence the necessity for them has been all but abolished. This is the outcome of strict rules, costly landfill fees, and an emphasis on trash minimization techniques.

Furthermore, Sweden's environmental awareness culture supports its waste management practices. The value of trash reduction and recycling is instilled in citizens from a young age. High levels of public involvement and a feeling of accountability for waste management have resulted from this.

The extended producer responsibility (EPR) theory, in which producers are responsible for all aspects of a product's lifespan, including appropriate disposal, is also highlighted by the Swedish model. This promotes the creation of more environmentally friendly goods and packaging.

Sweden's achievement in waste management and reduction is proof of the value of all-encompassing legislation, technological integration, and societal dedication to sustainability. Sweden has established a standard for other countries to follow in their quest for efficient waste management solutions by concentrating on waste-to-energy, efficient recycling, limited landfill use, and cultivating a culture of environmental responsibility.

Let's examine yet another effective case study of waste management and reduction, this time concentrating on Japan.

Japan has become well-known internationally for its cutting-edge waste management techniques and a high degree of trash reduction. Japan has evolved a diverse strategy for managing its trash because of its limited geographical area and high cultural focus on cleanliness and effectiveness.

The "3R" principle—reduce, reuse, and recycle—is one of Japan's prominent waste reduction techniques. The nation puts a high priority on decreasing trash at the source by encouraging producers to reduce packaging and advertise eco-friendly goods. Additionally, residents are urged to lead a minimalist lifestyle and make deliberate decisions that minimize trash production.

The recycling programs in Japan are some of the most sophisticated in the world. The nation has an efficient system for collecting and separating garbage. Residents must separate their trash into categories including hazardous garbage, recyclable materials, burnable materials, and non-burnable materials. This rigorous procedure of sorting makes recycling effective and lowers contamination of recyclable items.

Along with recycling, Japan also encourages the practice of "kuru-kuru recycling," sometimes known as "turn-turn recycling." This entails encouraging residents to recycle materials inside their own homes, including repurposing empty containers into shelving or planters. This strategy promotes creativity and motivates individuals to come up with innovative applications for things that might otherwise go to trash.

The waste-to-energy (WTE) plants in Japan are also very important for trash management. The nation has made significant investments in WTE technology to turn non-recyclable garbage into electricity due to the limited amount of accessible land. This lowers the amount of waste sent to landfills and helps create renewable energy.

The effectiveness of Japan's waste management system also heavily depends on public engagement and education. To increase public knowledge of garbage reduction, sorting, and appropriate disposal, the government and local communities collaborate. Waste management education is often included in the curriculum of schools, fostering positive habits from a young age.

In conclusion, Japan's waste management and reduction policies serve as an example of the nation's dedication to sustainability, effectiveness, and innovation. Japan has established itself as a worldwide pioneer in efficient waste management techniques via a mix of trash reduction at the source, painstaking sorting and recycling, waste-to-energy plants, and a strong focus on education and public participation.

Chapter Four

Towards Sustainable Solutions: Reducing Our Waste Footprint

The need to lessen our environmental impact has never been more important in an age marked by growing worries about resource depletion and environmental damage. The amount of garbage produced on a global scale has risen to worrisome levels, placing excessive stress on ecosystems, contaminating water supplies, and accelerating climate change. In response, communities and countries are adopting sustainable solutions in greater numbers that aim to reduce waste production, improve resource utilization, and promote a circular economy.

The maxim "Reduce, Reuse, Recycle" is at the heart of the movement to reduce waste. A sustainable waste management plan is built based on this trio. Promoting responsible consumption, pressuring manufacturers to provide items with little packaging, and implementing waste-reduction strategies are all steps in the process of reducing waste at the source. Reuse helps us increase product longevity and reduce the need for fresh materials. Recycling simultaneously reduces the requirement for raw material extraction and lessens the environmental effect of industrial operations by turning waste materials into marketable goods.

Furthermore, a paradigm change from a linear economy to a circular economy is required for sustainable waste reduction. To reduce waste creation, the circular economy concept proposes a closed-loop system in which goods and materials are made to be reused, mended, or recycled. Collaboration amongst industries is necessary for this strategy, from firms and governments to consumers and innovators. This joint effort is what gives the idea of extended producer responsibility (EPR) more recognition. EPR makes producers liable for the whole product lifespan and encourages eco-friendly design and ethical disposal procedures.

Achieving waste reduction targets depends in large part on technological innovation. The most effective use of resources is made possible through waste-to-energy (WTE) facilities, cutting-edge recycling technology, and digital systems for trash monitoring and management. In addition, cutting-edge technologies like bioplastics, which are made from renewable resources and degrade over time, provide viable substitutes for conventional plastics and help to address the challenge of plastic waste.

Campaigns for education and awareness are a crucial component of efforts to reduce waste. Promoting environmental literacy gives people the information and resources they need to make wise decisions, such as adopting zero-waste lifestyles or actively taking part in regional waste management programs. Such initiatives ensure the lifetime of waste reduction efforts by fostering a culture of accountability and stewardship.

In conclusion, finding sustainable ways to reduce our waste footprint requires a thorough and varied strategy. We can all work together to create a more sustainable future by adopting the concepts of reducing, reusing, and recycling, implementing a circular economy, encouraging technological advancement, and placing a high priority on education and awareness. Although the task is difficult, the advantages it might have for the environment, society, and future generations are immense.

The role of education and public awareness in waste management

To address the growing global trash challenge, education, and public awareness are vital to waste management. This strategy promotes sustainable practices and goes beyond the simple disposal of garbage to address its underlying causes. Education enables people to make educated decisions that have a direct influence on the environment by promoting understanding about waste reduction, recycling, and responsible consumption.

Effective waste management education begins in schools at a young age when kids are taught about the product life cycle, the effects of garbage on ecosystems, and the value of recycling. They are given the information necessary to critically assess their consuming habits and make informed choices thanks to this foundation. Additionally, waste management professionals may educate communities by holding lectures and seminars that emphasize the negative effects incorrect garbage disposal has on the environment and society.

Campaigns to raise public awareness reinforce the message. To reach a larger audience, these campaigns make use of a variety of media, including social media, television, and local events. They highlight the maxim "Reduce, Reuse, Recycle" and provide creative trash management techniques. These efforts alter cultural attitudes by making trash management a regular topic of discourse, elevating waste from a minor nuisance to a shared duty.

By putting into place rules that encourage responsible waste management, governments and local authorities play a crucial part in raising public awareness. Regulations requiring trash separation, mandated recycling programs, and campaigns encouraging the purchase of eco-friendly goods are a few examples of these policies. Such actions help the public adopt sustainable practices while also highlighting the significance of garbage management.

In the long term, public awareness and education help to transform culture's perspective on waste. People become more proactive in looking for ways to reduce waste output as they start to internalize the effects of their activities. As a result, the burden on landfills is lessened, and a circular economy where resources are preserved and repurposed is encouraged to expand.

Responsible Consumer Choices: Reducing Packaging and Single-Use Items

Making good buying decisions has become very important in the modern period when environmental issues are at the forefront. The deliberate attempt to minimize packaging waste and the usage of single-use goods is an essential component of this. This strategy involves spreading more sustainable practices throughout businesses and producers, not only encouraging individuals to make better choices for themselves.

When customers choose items with minimum or environmentally friendly packaging, manufacturers are forced to rethink their packaging strategy. This phenomenon could encourage the adoption of readily recyclable, compostable, or biodegradable materials and result in a change in industry standards. Additionally, it encourages creativity in package design, inspiring companies to come up with inventive solutions to safeguard goods while reducing their environmental impact.

The decision to purchase items with less packaging sends a message to companies that customers value sustainability. Companies may be motivated by this pressure to investigate packaging alternatives such as bulk dispensers, refill stations, and package-free choices. Additionally, it encourages the "bring your own container" philosophy, which eliminates the need for single-use packaging.

Speaking of single-use goods, there is a growing worldwide push to limit their use. Straws, cutlery, and coffee cups are just a few examples of single-use plastics that greatly increase waste and pollution. Customers drastically reduce their contribution to landfill and ocean garbage by choosing reusable alternatives like stainless steel straws, bamboo cutlery, and insulated travel mugs.

In the overall scheme of things, individual decisions matter more. Businesses note the change in demand as more consumers adopt reusable things and start to provide more sustainable solutions. Stores may urge consumers to bring their bags, while cafes and restaurants may convert to biodegradable utensils. Conscious consumer decisions drive systemic change as a result of these acts.

Furthermore, influencing legislative changes is directly correlated with informed consumer decisions about packaging and single-use goods. Governments and regulatory organizations are more likely to impose bans or limitations on certain single-use goods as a result of consumer demand for change. This is in line with the more general objective of environmental protection and waste minimization.

Finally, in the context of waste management, the influence of wise consumer decisions cannot be understated. Individuals influence improvements in business practices and political choices by choosing reusable goods and products with less packaging. By minimizing waste, preserving resources, and protecting the environment for future generations, we help to create a more sustainable future.

Collaboration between Industries, Governments, and Communities

Waste management is a difficult problem that needs a multifaceted solution. The development of efficient and long-lasting waste management systems is greatly aided by cooperation between businesses, governments, and local communities. Each party contributes special skills and resources to the table that, when combined, may provide useful answers.

By influencing manufacturing techniques and the materials utilized, industries have a significant influence on waste management. Industries may drastically minimize the trash produced at the source by using eco-friendly production techniques, developing goods with minimum packaging, and placing a high priority on recyclability. Industry may link its activities with more general sustainability aims by working with governments and communities.

On the other hand, governments have the authority to enact laws and regulations that direct waste management procedures. Governments provide a framework that encourages businesses and communities to abide by rules that support recycling, trash reduction, and appropriate disposal. They may also support extended producer responsibility (EPR) programs, in which producers take charge of product disposal and recycling. Such programs encourage businesses to develop goods with lifespan and the environment in mind.

Communities have a significant impact on garbage creation and disposal practices as end consumers. Promoting ethical consumption, trash separation, and recycling practices among communities via education and awareness campaigns. Additionally, communities provide crucial input to businesses and authorities on how well trash management programs are working. Their participation contributes to the development of policies and initiatives that are more useful and attentive to regional requirements.

Collaboration among these three parties creates a synergy that propels comprehensive transformation. Governments may provide incentives to businesses to follow sustainable practices, and businesses can fund neighborhood programs that encourage recycling and trash minimization. While simultaneously making businesses and governments responsible for their activities, communities gain from better waste management services and a healthier environment.

The creation of waste-to-energy technology is one illustrative example of effective teamwork. To reduce their dependency on landfills and provide a sustainable energy source, industries engage in research and innovation. Communities take part by separating garbage at the source and embracing the idea of energy recovery, while governments provide the necessary financing and regulatory assistance.

In conclusion, successful waste management policies are created via partnerships between businesses, governments, and communities. When these organizations collaborate, they make use of each other's advantages to promote systemic change. A more sustainable approach to waste management that benefits the environment and society at large is produced as a consequence of industry innovation, government regulation, and community adoption of ethical behavior.

Chapter Five

Shaping the Future: A World Beyond Trash

Visualize a future in which the concept of garbage is rendered obsolete—a society in which resources are preserved, exploited, and changed in ways that do away with the need for conventional waste disposal techniques. In this future, materials and goods are created with lifespan and recycling in mind, resulting in a paradigm change from a linear economy to a circular economy.

Innovative technologies are crucial in this newly reshaped environment. Modern techniques for sorting and recycling may effectively separate items for reuse, reducing the requirement to remove raw resources. A product may be simply dismantled and rebuilt thanks to 3D printing technology and the circular design principle, which lowers waste production and encourages repairability.

Additionally, biotechnology helps create a planet free of garbage. Utilizing microbes, organic waste may be broken down into useful products like compost or biofuels. To ensure that plastics, which have long been a problem, do not remain in the environment, they might be made to be biodegradable or even edible.

The change transcends mere elements, which is significant. Attitudes change as well. With the popularity of sharing and subscription models, the idea of ownership shifted. People value experiences more than things, which lowers the need for new goods and, as a result, lowers trash production.

In this future, sustainability prevails as the idea of rubbish is rethought. A world without waste isn't just a concept; it's a real-world made possible by people working together, cutting-edge technology, and a dedication to protecting the environment. Even if the path may be difficult, the possibility of a better, more wealthy future is within our reach.

Policy and Regulatory Changes: Encouraging Sustainable Practices in Waste Management

The sustainability of the environment and the reduction of the harmful effects of garbage on ecosystems and human health depend critically on effective waste management. Many nations have enacted legal and policy measures that support environmentally friendly waste management practices to accomplish this. These adjustments include a range of tactics, including encouraging proper disposal practices, increasing recycling, and lowering trash output. We may learn more about how these methods might produce beneficial results by looking at effective programs from other nations.

The waste management strategy in Sweden is one such instance. Sweden has put in place several measures that have produced an exceptional waste management system with high rates of recycling and little use of landfills. Implementing a "pay-as-you-throw" system, in which families are taxed depending on the quantity of rubbish they create, is one important option. People are encouraged to generate less garbage and recycle more as a result. Sweden also makes significant investments in facilities that burn non-recyclable garbage to produce electricity. This helps the nation achieve its objectives for renewable energy while also reducing the dependency on landfills.

Another excellent example is Japan, which had trouble managing trash since there wasn't much room for landfills and there were a lot of people living there. Japan responded by implementing a thorough garbage sorting and recycling program. garbage must be divided into several categories, such as recyclable, hazardous, burnable, and non-recyclable garbage. Effective recycling operations and less contamination in recyclable materials are the results of this rigorous sorting. Japanese society has a strong "3R" philosophy—Reduce, Reuse, Recycle—which further supports sustainability.

The waste management practices in Germany are equally noteworthy. In this nation, producers are in charge of how their goods, including packaging, are disposed of at the end of their useful lives. This has sparked product design innovation, encouraged the use of recyclable materials, and reduced the need for extra packing. Recycling rates for glass and plastic bottles have greatly risen as a result of Germany's bottle deposit system, which provides reimbursements for returned beverage containers.

The waste management practices in their various nations have been significantly impacted by these policies and legislative developments. Due to Sweden's emphasis on waste-to-energy and recycling, just 1% of the nation's garbage is now disposed of in landfills. Over 80% of Japan's plastic garbage may be recycled thanks to thorough sorting. The producer responsibility policy adopted in Germany has increased recycling rates for packaging and decreased littering.

These nations have achieved notable progress towards more effective and ecologically friendly waste management systems by promoting responsible trash disposal, recycling, and sustainable behaviors. These effective strategies may serve as an example for other countries looking to tackle their waste management issues and encourage sustainable practices.

Technological Advances in Waste Management

Modern waste management techniques have undergone a radical transformation as a result of technical breakthroughs, which have provided creative answers to the problems of trash creation, disposal, and environmental effects. These technical advancements cover a broad variety of topics, including recycling and trash-to-energy conversion as well as garbage collecting and sorting. These technological developments have a significant impact on changing the waste management environment as the globe looks for more sustainable solutions.

- **Smart Waste Collection Systems**

Traditional waste collection methods often result in inefficiencies, with garbage trucks following fixed routes regardless of fill levels. Sensors and data analytics are used in smart garbage collection systems to optimize routes and schedules based on real-time fill data. This not only lowers fuel use and pollutants but also guarantees prompt garbage collection. Cities like Barcelona and Singapore, for instance, have put such systems in place, which has resulted in cost savings and cleaner cities.

- **Automated Sorting Technologies**

Manual sorting of recyclable materials can be time-consuming and prone to errors. The accuracy and effectiveness of garbage sorting have significantly increased thanks to new sorting technologies including robotic arms and conveyor belt systems with sensors and cameras. These systems can recognize and classify various recyclable materials, reducing contamination and raising the value of recycled resources.

- **Plasma Gasification and Pyrolysis**

Plasma gasification and pyrolysis are sophisticated waste-to-energy techniques that turn waste materials into energy and useful byproducts. Waste is broken down into syngas by plasma gasification using high-temperature plasma arcs, which may then be utilized to create energy or chemicals. Pyrolysis is the process of heating garbage without oxygen to create char, gas, and oil. These innovations lessen trash production, decrease the need for landfill space, and aid in the production of renewable energy.

- **E-Waste Recycling Innovations**

The rapid growth of electronic waste (e-waste) presents unique challenges due to its complex composition. Innovative e-waste recycling technologies recover priceless metals and components from discarded electronics using processes including mechanical shredding, hydrometallurgical extraction, and microbiological procedures. These procedures lessen the need for virgin resources while also preventing the release of hazardous compounds into the environment.

- **Blockchain for Transparency**

Blockchain technology is being investigated to improve traceability and transparency in the supply chains for waste management. Blockchain technology may discourage unlawful dumping, encourage correct disposal, and guarantee that trash is handled by authorized parties by producing tamper-proof records of waste transactions and movements.

- **Waste analytics and predictive modeling**

To estimate the patterns of waste creation, data analytics, and predictive modeling technologies examine both historical and current data. This makes it possible for waste management organizations to allocate resources efficiently, prepare for times of increased trash production, and carry out focused recycling and collecting programs.

- **Biodegradable Packaging and Materials**

The creation of biodegradable packaging materials derived from plant-based sources is the result of technological developments. Natural decomposition of these materials lessens the negative environmental effects of single-use plastics and packaging trash.

- **Waste Reduction Apps and Platforms**

To promote and support waste reduction activities among people and organizations, mobile apps and digital platforms have evolved. These networks encourage the sharing and reuse of goods and give waste reduction advice and information on recycling drop-off locations.

These technological developments have a great deal of potential to improve trash management and make it more sustainable and ecologically friendly. Societies may aim to reduce waste creation, maximize resource recovery, and minimize the environmental effects related to garbage disposal by using smart systems, automation, inventive waste-to-energy technology, and data-driven initiatives. The potential to transform waste management procedures and contribute to a greener future is becoming more and more real as technology advances.

Cultivating Mindsets of Environmental Stewardship

To address the expanding issues with waste management and promote a sustainable future, it is essential to cultivate an attitude of environmental stewardship. This strategy emphasizes individual accountability, awareness, and proactive involvement in lowering waste production, increasing recycling, and supporting environmentally beneficial practices. Waste management may be improved by embedding these principles at the individual, local, and societal levels to make it more effective, efficient, and environmentally friendly.

- **Education and Awareness Campaigns**

Environmental stewardship starts with education. People may grasp the negative effects of irresponsible trash disposal and the advantages of responsible practices with the aid of educational programs and awareness campaigns. Schools, community organizations, and media sources are crucial in spreading knowledge about recycling, trash reduction, and the effects of garbage buildup on the environment.

- ## Promoting Behavior Change

Behavior must be influenced to change thoughts. Governments, corporations, and non-governmental organizations may work together to develop incentive-based initiatives that motivate people to develop sustainable waste management practices. Reward programs, like discounts for reusable goods or tax breaks for recycling, may inspire individuals to make thoughtful decisions.

- ## Engaging Communities

Developing a feeling of shared responsibility requires community participation. People may get together via seminars, recycling activities, and community clean-up efforts to solve waste-related issues in their communities. People are more likely to adopt sustainable practices if they interact with people who have similar ideals.

- ## Role of Businesses and Industries

Businesses and their industries play a big part in the trash-generating process via packaging and manufacturing methods. A culture of environmental stewardship may be promoted by encouraging companies to utilize eco-friendly packaging, reduce the use of single-use plastics, and develop effective trash disposal techniques. Initiatives in corporate social responsibility that place a high priority on waste reduction might motivate both clients and staff to adopt similar practices.

- **Incorporating Sustainability in Design**

Designers and architects may include sustainable ideas in their works. This entails utilizing materials that have a smaller environmental effect, creating readily recyclable goods, and taking into account a product's whole lifespan, from manufacture to disposal.

- **Technology and innovation**

Technology may significantly influence how people think. Gamification approaches, interactive platforms, and mobile applications may all be used to inform and involve people in waste reduction initiatives. Apps that monitor individual waste reduction targets or provide guidance on recycling techniques, for instance, may enable users to take control of their environmental effects.

- **Leadership and Role Models**

Political and community leaders, well-known people, and role models may use their platforms to promote recycling and environmental care. Their impact may encourage more people to engage in sustainable behaviors and see them as desirable behaviors.

- **Fostering Connection with Nature**

Maintaining a connection to nature may heighten one's feeling of responsibility. Environmental volunteerism, outdoor adventures, and enjoyment of nature are all activities that may help people develop a sense of the beauty of the earth and the need to conserve it.

- **Long-Term Thinking**

Environmental stewardship requires seeing beyond the present and taking activities' long-term effects into account. Even though they involve more work now, encouraging individuals to adopt decisions that support long-term sustainability may result in good mentality changes.

Waste management may change from being a reactive process to a proactive one by promoting an attitude of environmental care. Individuals contribute to a culture of sustainability when they start to see trash as a resource and understand their responsibility to reduce its effects. Societies may collaborate to develop a more responsible approach to waste management that benefits the environment and future generations via education, engagement, technology, and leadership.

Conclusion

The conclusion of "Beyond Trash: Rethinking Waste in the Modern World," the result of in-depth study and smart analysis, provides a compelling vision of a future where trash is not just a problem but also a solution ready to be harnessed. I deftly intertwine the complex strands of environmental science, society, and history to expose the false assumptions that have contributed to the present garbage issue.

The book explores the underutilized value of garbage as a resource with rigorous attention to detail, challenging preconceived beliefs and showing cutting-edge methods that change our connection with waste materials. The presented vision is both aspirational and anchored in practical tactics, which inspires readers to reevaluate their opinions on waste management and to push for change on both an individual and social level.

The foundation of the book's solution-focused approach is my proposal for a circular economy, in which items are made to be recycled and used for new purposes. The story persuadingly demonstrates how accepting this paradigm change may minimize environmental harm, lessen resource depletion, and stimulate unanticipated economic development by using examples from real-world situations and success stories.

"Beyond Trash" provides a vivid image of a society where garbage is no longer a gloomy weight but a wellspring of opportunity in this thought-provoking finale. It ends with a call to action that encourages readers to take an active role in the continuing conversation about trash management and environmental sustainability. The book serves as a light of hope, pointing us in the direction of a future where waste is not just a problem but also a driver of progress in contemporary society because of its thorough research, fresh viewpoints, and convincing arguments.

www.ingramcontent.com/pod-product-compliance
Lightning Source LLC
Chambersburg PA
CBHW050844260726

48660CB00006B/2429